DESIGN AND MANUFACTURE OF PHARMACEUTICAL TABLETS

DESIGN AND MANUFACTURE OF PHARMACEUTICAL TABLETS

REYNIR EYJOLFSSON

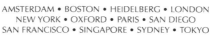

AMSTERDAM • BOSTON • HEIDELBERG • LONDON
NEW YORK • OXFORD • PARIS • SAN DIEGO
SAN FRANCISCO • SINGAPORE • SYDNEY • TOKYO

Academic Press is an Imprint of Elsevier

Academic Press is an imprint of Elsevier
32 Jamestown Road, London NW1 7BY, UK
525 B Street, Suite 1800, San Diego, CA 92101-4495, USA
225 Wyman Street, Waltham, MA 02451, USA
The Boulevard, Langford Lane, Kidlington, Oxford OX5 1GB, UK

Notices
Knowledge and best practice in this field are constantly changing. As new research and experience
broaden our understanding, changes in research methods, professional practices, or medical treatment
may become necessary.

Practitioners and researchers must always rely on their own experience and knowledge in evaluating
and using any information, methods, compounds, or experiments described herein. In using such
information or methods they should be mindful of their own safety and the safety of others, including
parties for whom they have a professional responsibility.

To the fullest extent of the law, neither the Publisher nor the authors, contributors, or editors, assume
any liability for any injury and/or damage to persons or property as a matter of products liability,
negligence or otherwise, or from any use or operation of any methods, products, instructions, or ideas
contained in the material herein.

British Library Cataloguing-in-Publication Data
A catalogue record for this book is available from the British Library.

Library of Congress Cataloging-in-Publication Data
A catalog record for this book is available from the Library of Congress.

ISBN: 978-0-12-802182-8

For information on all Academic Press publications
visit our website at http://store.elsevier.com/

This book has been manufactured using Print On Demand technology. Each copy is produced to order
and is limited to black ink. The online version of this book will show color figures where appropriate.

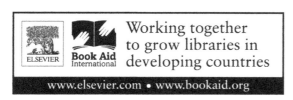

DEDICATION

This book is dedicated to my fellow pioneers at Pharmaco, Delta, and later Actavis, who laid the foundations to what Actavis is today: the third largest pharmaceutical generics company in the world.

CONTENTS

PREFACE

Many excellent books have been written about the design and manufacture of pharmaceutical tablets, but they are all more or less theoretical, offering few and limited examples of real-life formulations. Almost invariably, these examples lack information on processing details, stability (shelf life), dissolution, and bioavailability. In view of this, there is really a need for a book describing real-life practical examples that have been validated and researched as to bioavailability. These aspects frequently appear daunting to newcomers to tablet formulation science and even to experienced professionals. From this author's experience the conclusion is: "If only I had had a book on the practical aspects of these matters when I started my career in this field things would have been much easier and more satisfying."

This book is an attempt to improve on this situation by offering nine real-life tablet formulations and processing examples. In order to avoid conceivable commercial conflicts the identities of the active pharmaceutical ingredients (APIs) are not revealed but some of their physicochemical properties are disclosed.

Primarily, theoretical aspects are not dealt with in this book as they are readily available elsewhere. There is emphasis on design of experiments (DOE) but this is mostly restricted to practical examples. Also, mixing of pharmaceutical powders is given special attention. This author admits that his views may be in conflict with the practices generally employed in the pharmaceutical industry but he is of the opinion that if his approach to powder mixing were followed, problems with tablet content uniformity would be virtually nonexistent!

Best thanks to the wonderful staff at Elsevier Inc., particularly my editors, Ms. Kristine Jones and Ms. Molly McLaughlin, for their patience and never-failing help.

Hafnarfjordur, Iceland, July 2014
Reynir Eyjolfsson
reynirey@mmedia.is

ABBREVIATIONS

Al/Al	aluminum/aluminum
Al/PVC	aluminum/polyvinyl chloride
ANOVA	analysis of variance
API	active pharmaceutical ingredient
ASL	augmented simplex lattice
CCD	central composite design
CPDD	calcium phosphate dibasic dihydrate ($CaHPO_4 \cdot 2H_2O$)
CR	conventional release
CYC	cyclization
DC	direct compression
DF	degrees of freedom
DOE	design of experiments
HCl	hydrochloric acid
HDPE	high-density polyethylene
HPM	hypromellose
HYD	hydrolysis
LOD	loss on drying
MCC	microcrystalline cellulose
MSR	mixing–sieving–remixing
N	newton
NLT	not less than
NMT	not more than
RSM	response surface methodology
SM	sieving–mixing
SR	slow release
USP	United States Pharmacopeia
WG	wet granulation

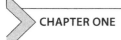

CHAPTER ONE

Introduction

1.1 GENERAL CONSIDERATIONS [1,2]

It has been stated that the discovery of new therapeutic entities always initiates excitement but even the best therapeutic entity in the world is of little value without an appropriate delivery system. The contributions of the formulation scientist are often either not well understood or taken for granted and thus remain unpraised. However, the drug entity and its delivery system cannot be separated.

Long time ago when this author entered into the realm of pharmacy the *Danish Pharmacopeia* (*Pharmacopoeia Danica 1948*) was official in Iceland. In it were numerous compositions and manufacturing methods for conventional pharmaceutical tablets. The formulations were practically always based on the same principle: lactose monohydrate was used as diluent and potato starch as diluent/disintegrant; granulation was done with gelatin mucilage as binder; the granulate was dried on trays, sieved, and lubricated with magnesium stearate/talc (1 + 9). These formulations were mostly compressed on single-punch tableting machines and did not generally suit high-speed rotaries. Tablets with poor technical properties were often obtained. Many pharmacies produced these tablets at the time, each using their own manufacturing "tricks." No direct compression tablets or slow-release tablets were in the pharmacopeia. Impurity testing, good manufacturing practices, and dissolution tests still lay in the future, more than a decade away.

Today, the majority of pharmaceutical tablets are still manufactured by wet granulation using a variety of binders and other excipients but the principles are the same as in the old days. When embarking on a new project of designing a generic tablet it is always desirable to ascertain which excipients the originator or other producers of generics use. This may save a lot of time in terms of compatibility studies. Information on this is now readily available on the Internet, e.g., at www.rxlist.com or www.medicines.org.uk, although quantitative data are not given there. During the years this author has used the *Repertorio Farmaceutico Italiano* and *L'Informatore Farmaceutico* (may be obtained from www.amazon.it) extensively, not only because of his fondness of the beautiful Italian language but

Design and Manufacture of Pharmaceutical Tablets. http://dx.doi.org/10.1016/B978-0-12-802182-8.00001-5

also because these sources furnished quantitative data of all ingredients in all pharmaceutical specialties registered in Italy. This practice, however, was abandoned some years ago. It is also highly recommended to screen the scientific literature about the chemical properties and perform functional group analysis of the active pharmaceutical ingredient's (API's) molecule in order to establish or at least be able to anticipate possible degradation pathways. Moreover, a particle size determination method for the API should be developed as soon as possible.

Knowledge of all excipients, even quantitatively, is not, of course, enough to immediately write down a proposal for an excellent tablet design/production method. What is gravely missing is information on how the ingredients are put together. It may even be difficult to determine whether the originator's tablet in question is manufactured by direct compression, wet or dry granulation. Occasionally, some information on this may be obtained from the patent literature (www.uspto.gov; www.epo.org) but in these cases another serious obstacle may be discovered, namely, the patent itself! Here, the formulation scientist's experience, creativity, and insight are crucial.

If a wet granulation method is selected, purified water is the preferred granulation liquid unless the API is very moisture sensitive, very hydrophobic, or presents special micromeritic properties (cf. Sections 2.5 and 3.3). In these cases ethanol 96% is advisable. Sometimes, ethanol 96%/ purified water (1 + 1) is used (cf. Section 2.3).

It is the experience of this author that the originator's formula can only very rarely be "copied" exactly. There are several reasons for this, e.g., unknown physical properties of API, unknown physical properties of excipients, and unknown manufacturing methods. Thus, the often heard remark that "copying" an existing formulation must be a simple matter is absolutely not true. The originator's list of excipients, even quantitative, most often only can serve as a reference model in development of a new formulation by varying the concentrations of the excipients in a systematic fashion following the principles of experimental design [design of experiments (DOE)]. Use of as few excipients as possible is essential. It is important to use similar equipment in small-scale experiments to those that will be used later in trial and production scale. Very good small-scale equipment for formulation development and processing is available, e.g., from the firm Procept (www.procept.be).

Finally a few words about tablet formulation/composition patents. These can be difficult to circumvent without infringement but may often be passed by using different excipients (see Section 2.3 for an example) or different production methods from those of the patent. Otherwise, it is the opinion of this author that the majority of these patents are not worth much in terms of novelty and he has often been surprised by the granting of patents based on procedures obvious to most persons skilled in the art!

1.2 PARTICLE SIZES [3]

The single most important physical parameter of a particulate API is unquestionably its particle size. As to tablets this variable may be expected to have impact on drug dissolution/bioavailability, content uniformity, and processability. Striking examples of the last subject are discussed in Sections 2.5 and 3.3.

Results of particle size measurements are very dependent on the experimental methodology. Unless the method used is described in detail particle measurement data are not of much value. The methods used in the pharmaceutical industry are sieving (mostly used on excipients), optical microscopy, and laser light diffraction.

Laser light diffraction is by far the most popular method as it is rapid, uses a large number of particles, and is very stable (robust). It involves dispersion of particles in air or in a liquid medium in which, of course, the sample must be insoluble. Laser light is beamed through the dispersion and the resulting diffracted light is detected on a system of sensors and transformed by appropriate mathematical procedures into a particle size distribution. This approach treats the particles as if they were perfect spheres, which, naturally, is practically never the case. Therefore, the results must be correlated with data obtained from optical and/or electron microscopy.

In optical microscopy the powder sample is spread on a glass slide and the particles inspected using a suitable magnification. This gives excellent information about particle shapes but it is not always easy to sort out primary particles from agglomerates. It is difficult and time consuming to get a statistically complete description of particle distributions by microscopy mainly due to small sample size, although computerized image analysis software is helpful.

The procedure for particle size distribution analysis by sieving (mostly used on excipients as stated above) is described in detail in the USP. This method requires a large amount of sample and is time consuming. Little information on "fines" is obtained.

1.3 EXCIPIENTS [4]

All particulate excipients mentioned in Chapters 2 and 3 are described here with emphasis on the properties pertinent to tablet design/technology.

1.3.1 Ac-Di-Sol SD-711

Croscarmellose sodium. Disintegrant, normally used in 2% concentration in tablets made by direct compression and 3% by wet granulation. White or grayish-white powder, practically insoluble in anhydrous ethanol. Hygroscopic. Insoluble in water but rapidly swells in it to four to eight times the original volume. Density in bulk 0.53 g/ml. pH 5–7 in an aqueous slurry. Loss on drying (LOD) NMT 10%, 105°C. Particle size data: NMT 2% retained on 200-mesh (74 μm) and NMT 10% on 325-mesh (45 μm) screen. Laser light diffraction specifications (dry powder?): d(10) NMT 25 μm, d(0.5) 25–55 μm, and d(0.9) NLT 60 μm.

1.3.2 Aerosil 200

Colloidal silicon dioxide. Glidant, antiadherent, used in 0.1–1% concentration. A light, fine, white amorphous powder. Practically insoluble in water. Hygroscopic. Density in bulk 0.03–0.04 g/ml. pH 3.7–4.7 in 4% aqueous dispersion. LOD NMT 1.5%, 105°C. Mean primary particle size 12 nm.

1.3.3 Avicel PH-102

Microcrystalline cellulose. Binder, diluent, used in 10–90% concentration. White or almost white, fine granular powder. Practically insoluble in water, in ethanol, and in dilute acids. Hygroscopic. Density in bulk 0.28–0.33 g/ml. pH 5.5–7.0 in aqueous dispersion. LOD 3.0–5.0%, 105°C. Mean nominal particle size 100 μm. NMT 8% retained on 60-mesh (250 μm) and NLT 45% on 200-mesh (75 μm) screen.

1.3.4 Compactrol

Calcium sulfate dihydrate. Diluent. White or off-white, free-flowing, fine granular powder. Very slightly soluble in water, practically insoluble in alcohol. Nonhygroscopic. Bulk density NMT 1.10 g/ml. We have found pH 6.8 in 20% aqueous slurries and LOD 0.2% at 80°C. Mean particle size 120 μm. NLT 85% retained on 140-mesh (100 μm) and NLT 98% pass through 40-mesh (425 μm) screen.

1.3.5 Corn starch

Maize starch. Binder, diluent, disintegrant. Matt, white to slightly yellowish, very fine powder that creaks when pressed between the fingers. Practically insoluble in cold water and in ethanol (96%). Bulk density 0.45–0.58 g/ml. pH 4.0–7.0 in 20% aqueous slurry. LOD NMT 15.0%, 130°C. Mean particle size 13 μm.

1.3.6 Di-Tab

Dibasic calcium phosphate dihydrate, dicalcium phosphate dihydrate, calcium hydrogen phosphate. Diluent, direct compression diluent. White, free-flowing, crystalline powder. Practically insoluble in cold water and in alcohol. Dissolves in dilute hydrochloric acid. Nonhygroscopic. May lose water of crystallization under certain conditions. Bulk density 0.95 g/ml. pH 7.4 in 20% aqueous slurry. We have found LOD 0.8% at 80°C. Mean particle size 180 μm. Particle size specifications: NMT 1% retained on 20-mesh (850 μm), NMT 2% retained on 40-mesh (425 μm), 40–80% retained on 100-mesh (150 μm), and NMT 5% pass through 325-mesh (45 μm) screen.

1.3.7 Eudragit RS PO

Ammonio methacrylate copolymer type B. Slow-release control agent independent of pH. Colorless to white or almost white, free-flowing, fine granular powder. Practically insoluble in water, freely soluble in ethanol. Tends to form lumps if stored above 30°C but this has no influence on quality; the lumps are easily broken up again. Density in bulk 0.39 g/ml. LOD NMT 3.0%, vacuum, 80°C. Particle size specification: NLT 90% pass through 315 μm screen.

1.3.8 Magnesium stearate 5712

Magnesium stearate Hyqual, magnesium stearate. Lubricant of vegetable origin used in 0.2–5% concentration, most commonly 0.5%. White, very fine, light powder, greasy to the touch. Practically insoluble in water and in ethanol. Bulk density 0.16 g/ml. LOD NMT 4.0%, 105°C. Sieve test: NLT 99.5% pass through 325-mesh (45 μm) screen. Particle size by laser light diffraction (dry powder?): d(0.5) 6–14 μm and d(0.9) NMT 35 μm.

1.3.9 Mannitol 60

Mannitol. Soluble sugar alcohol diluent used in 10–90% concentration. Does not interfere with amino groups in APIs, thus eliminating risk of

Maillard reaction. White to almost white, crystalline powder. Freely soluble in water, very slightly soluble in ethanol (96%). Density in bulk 0.43 g/ml. LOD NMT 0.3%, 105°C. Mean particle size 60 μm. Sieve test: NMT 10% retained on 60-mesh sieve (250 μm).

1.3.10 Methocel K4M Premium

Hypromellose 2208. Slow-release control agent used in 10–80% concentration. White, yellowish white, or grayish white powder. Practically insoluble in hot water and in ethanol. It dissolves in cold water giving a colloidal solution. Hygroscopic after drying. pH 5.5–8.0 in 2% aqueous solution. Viscosity 2,663–4,970 mPa s in 2% solution in water at 20°C. Bulk density 0.34 g/ml. LOD NMT 5.0%, 105°C. Sieve test (slow-release grade): through 40 mesh (425 μm) NLT 99.0%, through 100 mesh (150 μm) NLT 90.0%, and through 230 mesh (63 μm) 50.0–80.0%.

1.3.11 Methocel K100M Premium

Hypromellose 2208. Slow-release control agent used in 10–80% concentration. White, yellowish white, or grayish white powder. Practically insoluble in hot water and in ethanol. It dissolves in cold water giving a colloidal solution. Hygroscopic after drying. pH 5.5–8.0 in 2% aqueous solution. Viscosity 75,000–140,000 mPa s in 2% solution in water at 20°C. Bulk density 0.34 g/ml. LOD NMT 5.0%, 105°C. Sieve test (slow-release grade): through 40 mesh (425 μm) NLT 99.0%, through 100 mesh (150 μm) NLT 90.0%, and through 230 mesh (63 μm) 50.0–80.0%.

1.3.12 Methocel K100LV Premium

Hypromellose 2208. Slow-release control agent used in 10–80% concentration. White, yellowish white, or grayish white powder. Practically insoluble in hot water and in ethanol. It dissolves in cold water giving a colloidal solution. Hygroscopic after drying. pH 5.5–8.0 in 2% aqueous solution. Viscosity 80–120 mPa s in 2% solution in water at 20°C. Bulk density 0.34 g/ml. LOD NMT 5.0%, 105°C. Sieve test (slow-release grade): through 40 mesh (425 μm) NLT 99.0%, through 100 mesh (150 μm) NLT 90.0%, and through 230 mesh (63 μm) 50.0–80.0%.

1.3.13 Pharmatose 150M

Lactose monohydrate. Lactose is probably the most common diluent in tablets; used in 10–90% concentration. Cannot be used with APIs containing amino groups due to Maillard reaction. White or almost white, crystalline powder. Freely but slowly soluble in water, practically insoluble in ethanol (96%). Density in bulk 0.62 g/ml. LOD NMT 0.5%, 105°C. Sieve test: through 45 μm NMT 50%, through 100 μm NLT 70%, through 150 μm NLT 85%, and through 315 μm NLT 100%.

1.3.14 Polyplasdone XL-10

Crospovidone. Disintegrant used in 2–8% concentration. White or yellowish-white powder. Practically insoluble in water and in alcohol. Hygroscopic. Bulk density 0.32 g/ml. LOD NMT 5.0%, 105°C. Typical mean particle size 25–40 μm.

1.3.15 Povidone

Povidone K30. Binder used in 0.5–5% concentration. White or yellowish-white powder. Freely soluble in water and in ethanol (96%). Very hygroscopic. Bulk density 0.3–0.4 g/ml. pH 3.0–5.0 for 5% aqueous solution. LOD NMT 5.0%, 105°C. Typical particle sizes determined by sieving: 90% NLT 50 μm, 50% NLT 100 μm, and 5% NLT 200 μm.

1.3.16 Primojel

Sodium starch glycolate. Disintegrant used in 2–8% concentration. White or almost white, fine, free-flowing powder. Soluble in water giving a translucent, gel-like product. Very hygroscopic. Bulk density 0.81 g/ml. pH 5.5–7.5 for a 3.3% gel in water. LOD NMT 7%, 105°C. Particle size specification: NLT 95% through 230-mesh sieve (63 μm).

1.3.17 Pruv

Sodium stearyl fumarate. Lubricant used in 0.5–2% concentration. White or almost white, fine powder with agglomerates of flat, circular particles. Practically insoluble in water and in ethanol. It is less hydrophobic than magnesium stearate or stearic acid and has less of a retardant effect on drug dissolution than these lubricants. Density in bulk 1.11 g/ml. pH 8.3 in 5% aqueous solution at 90°C. Water content NMT 5.0% (Karl Fischer). Particle size about 5–10 μm.

1.3.18 Sodium bicarbonate

Buffering agent, stabilizer. A white, crystalline powder. Soluble in water, practically insoluble in alcohol. Density in bulk 0.87 g/ml. pH 8.3 for a freshly prepared aqueous solution at 25°C.

1.3.19 Starch 1500

Pregelatinized starch. Binder, diluent, disintegrant typically used in 5–20% concentration. White or yellowish-white, free-flowing, fine granular powder. Swells in cold water, practically insoluble in alcohol. Hygroscopic. Bulk density 0.61 g/ml. pH 4.5–7.0 in 3% aqueous solution. LOD 7–9%, 105°C. Low water activity (0.33). Mean nominal particle size 65 μm. NLT 90% pass through 100-mesh screen (149 μm) and NMT 0.5% are retained on 40-mesh screen (420 μm).

1.3.20 Stearic acid 2236

Stearic acid. Lubricant of vegetable origin used in 1–3% concentration. White or yellowish-white, fine powder. Practically insoluble in water, soluble in alcohol. Density in bulk 0.55 g/ml. Practically no water content. Particle size specifications: 99–100% through 30-mesh (600 μm) and 95–100% through 100-mesh (150 μm) sieve.

1.3.21 Sterotex K

Hydrogenated vegetable oil. Lubricant and lipophilic slow-release control agent. White, fine powder. Practically insoluble in water. Melting point about 83°C. LOD NMT 0.1%, 105°C. Particle size specifications: NLT 99% through 40-mesh (425 μm) and NLT 95% through 100-mesh (150 μm) screen.

1.3.22 Tablettose 80

Lactose monohydrate. Agglomerated diluent for direct compression tableting. Cannot be used with APIs containing amino groups due to Maillard reaction. White or almost white, free-flowing, granular powder. Freely but slowly soluble in water, practically insoluble in ethanol (96%). Density in bulk 0.62 g/ml. LOD NMT 0.5%, 105°C. Particle size distribution: through 63 μm screen NMT 20%, through 180 μm screen 40–75%, through 400 μm screen NLT 85%, and through 630 μm screen NLT 97%.

1.3.23 Talc

Lubricant, glidant. A light, homogenous, white or almost white powder, greasy to the touch. Practically insoluble in water and in ethanol (96%). pH 7–10 in 20% aqueous slurry. Typical sieve analysis: NLT 99% through 325-mesh screen (44 μm).

1.4 EQUIPMENT

All mixing/granulating operations in production scale as described in Chapters 2 and 3 were performed with 150 l Collette (Collette-150) intensive mixer/granulator. Supposedly, other similar equipment may also be used, particularly if mixer blade tip speed is taken into account.

Sieving procedures were carried out with a Quadro Comil conical-type sieving machine or an Apex hammer/knife comminuting mill. Similar machines may also be used, e.g., Fitzmill hammer/knife mills.

Drying of granulates was done in Freund VFC-60 (220 l) fluid bed dryer. It is also believed that similar equipment may be used.

Tablet compaction was usually done with the old workhorses Manesty B3B or Manesty Betapress. It may safely be stated that since these machines could be used any other tableting machine may be used!

Measurements of flowability were performed with a Flodex flow meter and express the minimum diameter (in millimeters) of the circular hole required for powder flow – thus, smaller values are better.

Determinations of LOD were done with Mettler HG-53 halogen moisture analyzer.

The most important parameter in industrial tablet manufacture is the formulation. A good formulation may be processed with almost any type of equipment.

Further information on these and similar machines/instruments may easily be obtained from the Internet – a mere few clicks away.

1.5 MIXING OF PHARMACEUTICAL POWDERS [5]

Appropriate mixing of solid particulate ingredients (powders) in tablet manufacture is of great importance in order to ensure a high-quality product having consistently a good/excellent content uniformity, not only of the API but also of all components in the formulation.

Mixing of tablet ingredients is almost always accompanied with sieving, the main purpose of the latter being elimination/reduction of agglomerates in the raw materials since most ordinary mixing equipment is unable to decompose them during mixing. It can safely be stated that most APIs are fine or very fine powders that are more or less prone to agglomeration and that several excipients possess this property also, even direct compression materials.

It appears to be a common practice in the pharmaceutical industry to start a mixing operation by sieving the raw materials separately followed by mixing in a suitable mixer. This approach, however, must be considered to be very questionable since materials that tend to agglomerate will rapidly reagglomerate after sieving, thus nullifying the benefits of the sieving operation. By contrast, mixing of the ingredients followed by sieving and remixing will in most cases effectively prevent the presence of agglomerates in the finished blend due to the simultaneous intermixing of all ingredients affected by this method. Additionally, since the APIs are frequently with the smallest particle sizes of the components, this procedure promotes the formation of ordered mixtures.

The above considerations generally apply to "ordinary" materials, i.e., those consisting of very fine or fine particles [approximately 20–100 (or 200) μm]. Some substances, e.g., micronized (particle size less than about 20 μm), highly cohesive or coarse materials, may demand special sieving/mixing/milling methods. Elaborate procedures may also be necessary with formulations containing ingredients in very small amounts (less than about 1%).

The following example is given to illustrate the importance of the positioning of the sieving step in mixing operations. In this case the goodness of mixing could simply be estimated visually, thus eliminating uncertainties possibly arising from demixing in sampling or handling of samples and/or analytical errors.

A total of 3,750 g pregelatinized starch, 250 g silicon dioxide colloidal, and 400 g red iron oxide were sieved separately through a 0.5 mm screen (Comil) and mixed for 5 min in a 25 l intensive mixer (Collette). This is called the premix.

A total of 2,125 g hypromellose, 2,125 g sodium bicarbonate, 3,750 g pregelatinized starch, 5,000 g API, 46,500 g lactose monohydrate, 250 g silicon dioxide colloidal, and 15,500 g microcrystalline cellulose were sieved separately through a 1.0 mm screen (Comil) and mixed with the premix in a 300 l tumbling mixer (GEI IBC) at 12 rpm for 17 min.

Visual inspection of the resulting blend revealed the presence of numerous white agglomerates in the powder bed. Consequently, the blend was sieved through a 1.0 mm screen (Comil) followed by mixing at 12 rpm for 5 min in the tumbling mixer. No agglomerates could be detected visually in the resulting mixture.

These findings unambiguously demonstrate that sieving the ingredients separately prior to mixing did not prevent the presence of agglomerates in the resulting powder mixture, whereas subsequent sieving and remixing eliminated them completely. Therefore, it was proposed that mixing all the ingredients followed by sieving and remixing would solve the problem and this prediction was fully confirmed in further trials.

In conclusion, based on long experience with hundreds of formulations, it is the firm opinion of this author that the method of "mixing–sieving–remixing" (MSR) tablet components outperforms the "sieving–mixing" (SM) approach by far. Using suitable production equipment the MSR technique is not much more labor intensive, and, importantly, it generally furnishes a high degree of confidence in reproducibly manufacturing high-quality products with good or excellent content uniformity.

1.6 DESIGN OF EXPERIMENTS [6–9]

1.6.1 Introduction to statistical design of experiments – the two-level factorial

1.6.1.1 Introduction

It has been remarked that the situation of the experimenter is often similar to that of a person attempting to map the depth of the sea by making soundings at a limited number of places. With restrictions on resources and time it is essential that a maximum of information is extracted from as few experiments as possible. The statistical approach is highly effective for this purpose. However, it should be strongly emphasized that this methodology is no substitute for a sound subject matter knowledge, creativity, and insight. On the other hand, a proper joint application of these factors improves the chances of successfully resolving a given developmental problem with the least experimental effort.

Statistically designed experiments were originally introduced in agricultural field trials more than 90 years ago and have been employed in industry for approximately 60 years. Somewhat later, these methods have found their way into pharmaceutical formulation research.

Many types of statistically designed experiments exist and the literature describing them including the statistical mathematical theory is large. Consequently, it is merely possible to touch the surface here. The following elementary account will mainly be concerned with only one type of designed experiments, but perhaps the most useful one: the two-level factorial.

1.6.1.2 Designed experiments

Most development projects involve:

Sorting out from many variables the important ones

Obtaining understanding of how variables affect product properties and thereby discovering how to change them or finding a better combination of them in order to accomplish a better result

These problems may be resolved by experimentation and one of the characteristics of the statistical methodology is preplanning or a structured approach. A designed experiment is a series of trials encompassing:

Planning by competent persons

Setting of targets for specific goals

Inclusion of all relevant variables

Sufficient number of experiments in order to detect important effects and eliminate trivial ones

Arrangement in a pattern that gives as much information as possible

1.6.1.3 Basic considerations

Averages are more stable than single observations. The reliability (goodness) of an averaged result depends on the number (n) of items averaged and follows approximately the square root of n. When comparing the effects of two different levels of an independent variable the averages are used as shown in Fig. 1.1. In Fig. 1.1a it is obvious that the level of the independent variable A has an effect on the dependent variable (response) Y. By contrast, the outcome is not so clear-cut in Fig. 1.1b and c.

Naturally, it is of much importance to determine whether a given variable (factor) has a real effect on a pertinent response or not. If a real effect of A on Y is mistakenly declared, a Type I error has been committed. On the other hand, a Type II error is made if detection of a real effect has failed.

Three main methods are employed to defend against both kinds of errors. The first concerns the number of experiments (n) to be run. According to statistical theory n should be ca. $16 \times (sd)^2/D^2$ at each level of the variable (A) in question. In this expression sd is the standard deviation of the response (Y) and D the possible real difference in the responses (Y) resulting from varying ($-/+$) the variable (A).

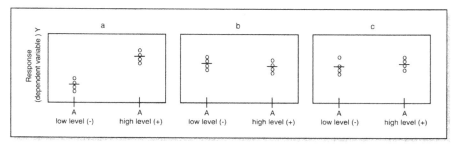

Figure 1.1 Influence of an independent variable on a dependent variable.

As a rule of thumb the number of experiments in two-level factorial designs should be at least 8 (4 at each level), but naturally this depends on the actual values of sd, D, and the number of variables (factors). Most practical projects require 4–32 experiments.

The second is utilization of a suitable statistical significance test to compare the results (responses) of the experiments. In this respect analysis of variance (ANOVA) and regression are prominent. The level of significance is usually set at $p < 0.05$.

The third technique is randomization, which means that the experiments and the subsequent analyses of them must be carried out randomly. This is very important in order to guarantee inferential validity in the face of unspecified, frequently time-related, disturbances, a major source of error. Unfortunately, however, randomization has frequently been neglected in scientific research resulting in dubious or false conclusions.

1.6.1.4 Two-level factorials

As a first simple example the possible effects of solids content (concentration) (A) and drying temperature (B) on the viscosity (stiffness) of a gel were investigated. As outlined above it would seem that this required running 16 experiments (4 for each level for 2 variables: $4 \times 2 \times 2 = 16$). However, inspection of Fig. 1.2a and b shows that eight experiments are sufficient since each experiment is actually used twice. That is, two variables (factors) can be studied in only eight trials. This is a 2^2-factorial with two replicates. The two-factor space is two-dimensional as depicted in Fig. 1.2c showing the responses (viscosity) at the corners of a rectangle.

Another display of the levels is shown in Table 1.1, which is a design matrix illustrating all the possible combinations arranged in standard order using coded units $(-/+)$ of the variables. Note the interaction column AB,

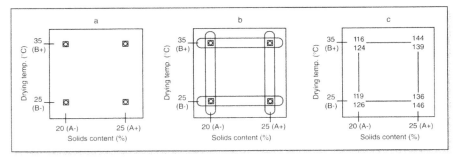

Figure 1.2 Effects of drying temperature and concentration on gel viscosity.

Table 1.1 Design matrix for the effects of drying temperature and concentration on gel viscosity

Standard order	A	B	AB	Response (stiffness rating)	
1	−	−	+	119	126
2	+	−	−	136	146
3	−	+	−	116	124
4	+	+	+	144	139
Effect	20	−1	1.5		
A: solids content (%)			B: drying temperature (°C)		
−	+		−	+	
20	25		25	35	

which is computed by multiplication of the corresponding signs $(-/+)$ in columns A and B. The purpose of the interaction term AB is to examine whether the effect of variable A depends on variable B or vice versa. Finally, the effects of the two variables and the interaction are given in the table. These are the differences between the high $(+)$ and low $(-)$ response data. Hence, the effects are calculated by associating the column signs with the response column, and then summing and dividing the sum by 4 as shown in the sequel.

A (solids content):

$$\text{Effect} = \frac{-119 - 126 + 136 + 146 - 116 - 124 + 144 + 139}{4} = 20$$

B (drying temperature):

$$\text{Effect} = \frac{-119 - 126 - 136 - 146 + 116 + 124 + 144 + 139}{4} = -1$$

AB (solids–temperature interaction):

$$\text{Effect} = \frac{+119 + 126 - 136 - 146 - 116 - 124 + 144 + 139}{4} = 1.5$$

The interpretation of these results is that the solids content (concentration) has a conspicuous and positive effect on the viscosity rating, whereas the effects of both drying temperature and the interaction are negligible or nonexistent. Statistical analysis by ANOVA confirms this: $F = 38.25$, probability $> F = 0.0008$.

Further experimentation with the gel can therefore be confined to variation of the solids content only in order to attain the desired viscosity quality.

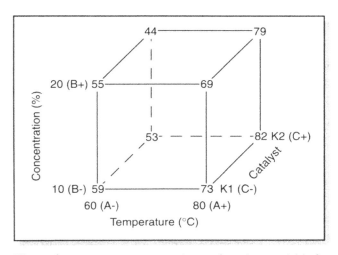

Figure 1.3 Effects of temperature, concentration, and catalyst on yield of synthesis.

The following two examples are borrowed from the field of chemical syntheses and are primarily intended as illustrations of the two-level factorial method. Of course, this methodology could be used to investigate, e.g., the levels of binder, disintegrant, lubricant, or glidant in a tablet formulation.

The second example deals with the results of a study aimed at maximizing the yield of a drug synthesis. Three variables were monitored, viz. reaction temperature (A), concentration (B), and type of catalyst (C). Running eight experiments is sufficient to ensure a fourfold replication of each of the effects since all the responses are used to supply information on each of them as shown in Fig. 1.3. This is a 2^3-factorial without replication. The three-factor space is three-dimensional (cf. Fig. 1.3): the responses (yields) are located at the corners of a cube.

Table 1.2 exhibits the design matrix including responses, main effects (A, B, C), and interaction effects (AB, AC, BC, ABC). The calculation of all effects is given below.

A (temperature):

$$\text{Effect} = \frac{-59 + 73 - 55 + 69 - 53 + 82 - 44 + 79}{4} = 23$$

B (concentration):

$$\text{Effect} = \frac{-59 - 73 + 55 + 69 - 53 - 82 + 44 + 79}{4} = -5$$

Table 1.2 Design matrix for the effects of temperature, concentration, and catalyst on the yield of a synthesis

Standard order	A	B	C	AB	AC	BC	ABC	Response (yield, %)
1	−	−	−	+	+	+	−	59
2	+	−	−	−	−	+	+	73
3	−	+	−	−	+	−	+	55
4	+	+	−	+	−	−	−	69
5	−	−	+	+	−	−	+	53
6	+	−	+	−	+	−	−	82
7	−	+	+	−	−	+	−	44
8	+	+	+	+	+	+	+	79
Effect	23	−5	0.5	1.5	9	−1	1.5	

A: temperature (°C)		B: concentration (%)		C: catalyst	
−	+	−	+	−	+
60	80	10	20	K1	K2

C (catalyst):

$$\text{Effect} = \frac{-59 - 73 - 55 - 69 + 53 + 82 + 44 + 79}{4} = 0.5$$

AB (temperature–concentration interaction):

$$\text{Effect} = \frac{+59 - 73 - 55 + 69 + 53 - 82 - 44 + 79}{4} = 1.5$$

AC (temperature–catalyst interaction):

$$\text{Effect} = \frac{+59 - 73 + 55 - 69 - 53 + 82 - 44 + 79}{4} = 9$$

BC (concentration–catalyst interaction):

$$\text{Effect} = \frac{+59 + 73 - 55 - 69 - 53 - 82 + 44 + 79}{4} = -1$$

ABC (temperature–concentration–catalyst interaction):

$$\text{Effect} = \frac{-59 + 73 + 55 - 69 + 53 - 82 - 44 + 79}{4} = 1.5$$

Inspection of the data reveals a negative concentration effect and a large positive temperature–catalyst interaction effect. Since temperature and catalyst are involved in an interaction no statement can be made about their individual effects: their effects must be considered jointly because the effect of each variable depends on the level of the other (cf. Fig. 1.3). The interaction evidently arises from a difference in sensitivity to temperature change for the two catalysts. In order to maintain hierarchy (i.e., ancestral lineage of effects flowing from main effects down through higher-order interactions) in the ANOVA analysis all four effects (A, B, C, and AC) must be included. This furnishes $F = 86.63$ and probability $> F = 0.0020$, i.e., a highly significant result. It appears to be a good strategy to increase reaction temperature while using catalyst K2 and holding concentration at 10% in order to augment the yield further.

1.6.1.5 Two-level fractional factorials

The two examples already described were full factorial designs, i.e., permitting complete analysis of all effects, main and interactions. The number of experimental runs required by a full 2^k-factorial setup increases geometrically with k. Thus, 4, 5, 6, and 7 factors (variables) demand 16, 32, 64, and 128 runs, respectively. Evidently, the experimental burden may become troublesome when dealing with many factors. Fortunately, it turns out that when k is not small the desired information may often be obtained by carrying out only a fraction of the full design. The reason for this is that there tends to be a redundancy in the design when k is not small. Analysis of, e.g., the full 7-factor design yields 128 statistics giving estimates of the following effects (AVG: average, ME: main effect, FI: factor interaction):

Effects	AVG	ME	2-FI	3-FI	4-FI	5-FI	6-FI	7-FI
Number	1	7	21	35	35	21	7	1

Although all these effects can be estimated, it does not imply that they are all of appreciable magnitude. There is a tendency in terms of absolute magnitude that main effects are larger than two-factor interactions (2-FI), 2-FI larger than 3-FI, etc. Generally, 3-FI tend to be small and 4-FI and higher-order interactions negligible. Also, it is frequently true when dealing with many variables that some of them have no detectable effect whatever. Fractional factorial analysis exploits these facts.

Table 1.3 presents the design matrix and the results of an investigation directed at optimizing the yield of a liquid-phase drug intermediate synthesis. Since there are 4 variables, a full design would require running 16 experiments. This has been reduced to eight, i.e., a half-fraction. The matrix was constructed by first arranging the first three factors (A, B, C) in standard order and then multiplying their signs in succession to furnish the signs

Table 1.3 Design matrix for effects of catalyst amount, temperature, pressure, and concentration on yield of a synthesis

Standard order	A BCD	B ACD	C ABD	D ABC	AB CD	AC BD	AD BC	Response (yield, %)
1	−	−	−	−	+	+	+	71
2	+	−	−	+	−	−	+	50
3	−	+	−	+	−	+	−	89
4	+	+	−	−	+	−	−	82
5	−	−	+	+	+	−	−	59
6	+	−	+	−	−	+	−	61
7	−	+	+	−	−	−	+	87
8	+	+	+	+	+	+	+	78
Effect	−8.75	23.75	−1.75	−6.25	0.75	5.25	−1.25	

A: catalyst amount (g)		B: temperature (°C)		C: pressure (atm)		D: concentration (%)	
−	+	−	+	−	+	−	+
10	15	220	240	3	5	10	12

of the fourth column (D). Following this, assignment of signs to the three remaining columns was performed as outlined in the first example above.

The full design would furnish determination of all main effects and interactions, that is:

A B C D (four ME)

AB AC AD BC BD CD (six 2-FI)

ABC ABD ACD BCD (four 3-FI)

$ABCD$ (one 4-FI)

Inevitably, the half-fractioning results in loss of information, viz. confounding or aliasing of the effects: The main effects are confounded with the effects of the three-factor interactions and the two-factor interactions with each other as depicted in the table. This fact signals that caution must be exercised in interpretation of the results.

The data indicate factors A (amount of catalyst), B (temperature), and D (concentration) as significant since the effects of the three-factor interactions would probably be small. The interaction effect requires more careful consideration: an interaction between A (amount of catalyst) and C (pressure) is unlikely since the synthesis is carried out in liquid phase. By contrast, interaction between B (temperature) and D (concentration) is probable judged by chemical reasoning. Further trials substantiated these assumptions.

It can be seen that the two-level factorials are primarily screening methods aimed at sorting out the significant factors from the trivial ones.

1.6.2 Response surface methodology (RSM)

1.6.2.1 Introduction

RSM encompasses a series of mathematical/statistical techniques for empirical model building and exploitation of the model. By means of appropriate design and analysis of experiments, RSM seeks to relate a response to the levels of a number of input variables or factors that influence it.

The two-level factorial designs are linearly modeled and therefore the resulting response surfaces in three-dimensional space are flat planes or, in the case of interactions, twisted planes (cf. the last section). Curvature in a response surface may be monitored by adding a center point into the two-factorial setup. If a significant curvature is detected, the next step might be running of smaller designs within the existing levels or to employ RSM.

It is repeated here that the two-level factorial designs are primarily screening methods employed to sort out the significant input variables in a given project. In many cases this may also be sufficient for optimization purposes. However, response surfaces frequently exhibit significant curvature. In these cases application of RSM may be the best approach.

The following elementary treatise will primarily be concerned with description of two examples: the first deals with analysis of a sieving process study involving two variables by RSM. The second illustrates the influence of three excipients in mixture in a direct compression tablet formulation, a special case of RSM.

1.6.2.2 RSM and a sieving process variable study

Many types of RSM designs exist but the most commonly utilized by far is the central composite design (CCD) (see Fig. 1.4, which illustrates the setup for two variables). For more factors the principle is similar. This design is a direct extension of the two-level factorial as shown by the four points labeled F. The levels are given in coded units. In addition to these there are five points: one center point (C) and four axial points (A). All points except the center point are located equidistantly on a circle with radius $\sqrt{2}$ (=1.414 = α). This endows the CCD with the highly desirable properties of orthogonality and rotatability.

Compared with two-level factorials the analysis of CCDs is more complicated and involves fitting of the experimental results with mathematical models by multiple linear regression. These polynomial models are displayed in Scheme 1.1. Additionally, computation of several statistics is necessary to assist in selecting the most appropriate model.

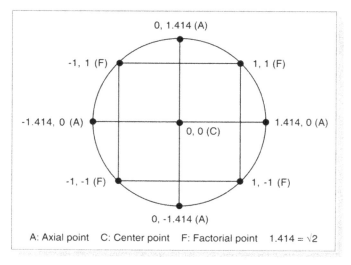

Figure 1.4 Central composite design setup for two variables.

Polynomials used for response surface designs:

Linear: $\eta = \beta_0 + \sum\limits_{i=1}^{q} \beta_i x_i$

Quadratic: $\eta = \beta_0 + \sum\limits_{i=1}^{q} \beta_i x_i + \sum\limits_{i=1}^{q}\sum\limits_{j=1}^{q} \beta_{ij} x_i x_j$

Cubic: $\eta = \beta_0 + \sum\limits_{i=1}^{q} \beta_i x_i + \sum\limits_{i=1}^{q}\sum\limits_{j=1}^{q} \beta_{ij} x_i x_j + \sum\limits_{i=1}^{q}\sum\limits_{j=1}^{q}\sum\limits_{k=1}^{q} \beta_{ijk} x_i x_j x_k$

Polynomials used for mixture designs (Scheffe-type):

Linear: $\eta = \sum\limits_{i=1}^{q} \beta_i x_i$

Quadratic: $\eta = \sum\limits_{i=1}^{q} \beta_i x_i + \sum\limits_{i<j}^{q}\sum\limits_{j=1}^{q} \beta_{ij} x_i x_j$

Special cubic: $\eta = \sum\limits_{i=1}^{q} \beta_i x_i + \sum\limits_{i<j}^{q}\sum\limits_{j=1}^{q} \beta_{ij} x_i x_j + \sum\limits_{i<j}\sum\limits_{j<k}\sum\limits_{k=1}^{q} \beta_{ijk} x_i x_j x_k$

Full cubic: $\eta = \sum\limits_{i=1}^{q} \beta_i x_i + \sum\limits_{i<j}^{q}\sum\limits_{j=1}^{q} \beta_{ij} x_i x_j + \sum\limits_{i<j}^{q}\sum\limits_{j=1} \delta_{ij} x_i x_j (x_i - x_j) + \sum\limits_{i<j}\sum\limits_{j<k}\sum\limits_{k=1}^{q} \beta_{ijk} x_i x_j x_k$

Scheme 1.1

Table 1.4 Design matrix for effects of sieve size and mill speed on tablet mass cv

Standard order	Sieve size (mm)		Mill speed (rpm)		Response (tablet mass cv, %)
	Coded	Actual	Coded	Actual	
1	−1	1.3	−1	985	0.77
2	1	2.7	−1	985	0.47
3	−1	1.3	1	2,240	0.29
4	1	2.7	1	2,240	0.45
5	−1.414	1.0	0	1,612	0.55
6	1.414	3.0	0	1,612	0.46
7	0	2.0	−1.414	725	0.66
8	0	2.0	1.414	2,500	0.31
9	0	2.0	0	1,612	0.50
10	0	2.0	0	1,612	0.47
11	0	2.0	0	1,612	0.51
12	0	2.0	0	1,612	0.46
13	0	2.0	0	1,612	0.48

Table 1.4 depicts the design layout and responses of a study aimed at minimizing tablet mass variation as measured by the coefficient of variation (cv) by varying the speed and screen size of a comminuting mill used for sieving of the parent granulate. All the milling experiments were performed in randomized order on aliquots of the same batch of granulate. Tablet compression was also carried out randomly by the same operator and on the same machine using identical compaction settings. Moreover, the tablet mass variation analyses were done in a randomized manner.

The center point (0, 0 in coded units) was replicated five times in order to estimate curvature, experimental ("pure") error, and lack of fit in the statistical analysis. All the other 8 points were nonreplicated, resulting in a total of 13 trials in the investigation.

The results of the statistical model fitting are summarized in Table 1.5. A brief explanation of the terms and their meaning in the present context follows:

ANOVA: Must be significant ($p > F$ less than 0.05).

Lack of fit: The variation of mean responses about the fitted model. Should be insignificant ($p > F$ larger than 0.10 is good).

Pred. R^2: Predicted R-squared. A measure of the amount of variation in new data explained by the model. Higher values are better.

PRESS: Predicted residual sum of squares. A measure of how well the model fits each point in the design. Smaller values are better.

Table 1.5 Results of statistical model fitting

Model	ANOVA		Lack of fit			
	F	p > F	F	p > F	Pred. R²	PRESS
Linear	11.97	0.0022	20.81	0.0055	0.3604	0.12
Quadratic	149.64	<0.0001	0.018	0.9961	0.9848	0.002854
Cubic	Aliased – too few unique design points to determine all terms in this model					

It is immediately evident from the above criteria that the quadratic model must be selected as the best approximation of the *true* response surface. By design, the CCD does not allow for determination of all terms in the cubic model but this is not of any concern here.

The resulting response surface is displayed in two-dimensional form (contour plot) in Fig. 1.5 and in three-dimensional view in Fig. 1.6.

The most striking result of a CCD RSM investigation is *the complete mapping of the response surface*, permitting estimation of a particular response

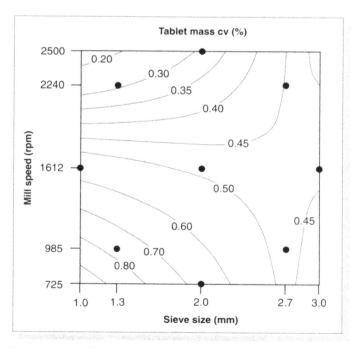

Figure 1.5 Response surface in two-dimensional form.

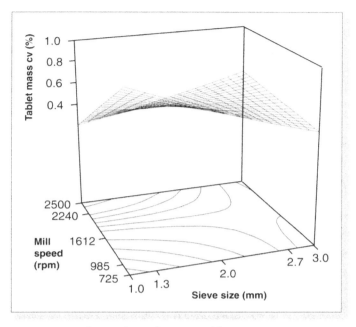

Figure 1.6 Response surface in three-dimensional form.

at all points within the design space. In this case the minimum tablet mass variation is found when high milling speeds and small–diameter sieve sizes are used for milling of the parent granulate. The optimum is near 2,240 rpm and 1.3 mm furnishing tablet mass cv of about 0.3%. Areas outside the design space should be considered with caution since this involves extrapolation of the model. In view of this, the point 2,500 rpm/1.0 mm showing a cv of less than 0.2% is hardly realistic. Besides, such low cv values are seldom attainable in practice using contemporary tableting technology.

1.6.2.3 RSM investigation of the properties of a three-component tablet formulation

RSM of mixtures represents a separate group due to loss of one degree of freedom (DF) since the proportion of all ingredients in mixtures always totals to unity. Hence, special polynomial models must be used for mixtures and these are detailed in Scheme 1.1. The most conspicuous difference between the polynomials for ordinary RSM and mixture models is absence of the intercept (β_0) in the latter arising from the DF constraint mentioned above.

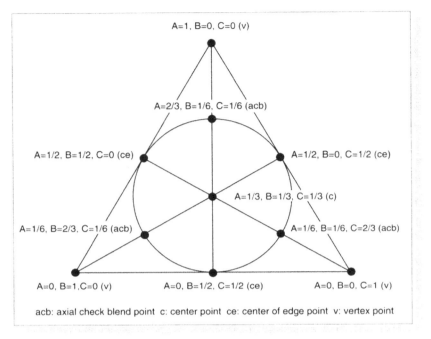

Figure 1.7 Augmented simplex lattice for three components.

It follows that the variable spaces for mixtures with two, three, and four components are a line, a triangle, and a tetrahedron, i.e., one-, two-, and three-dimensional, respectively. The corresponding response surfaces are two-, three-, and four-dimensional.

There are several types of mixture designs and one of the best is the augmented simplex lattice (ASL). This is displayed in Fig. 1.7 for three components. The simplex lattice proper is represented by six points, viz. the three vertex points plus the three center-of-edge points. Addition of four points in the interior area, i.e., one center point and three axial check points, affords the augmentation. The levels are given in pseudo-units (0–1), which are equivalent to the coded units of ordinary factorials (RSM). Inspection of the geometry of the ASL in Fig. 1.7 reveals that this arrangement furnishes the best possible distribution of design points within the experimental region.

Table 1.6 enumerates the design layout and responses from an investigation of a three-component direct compression tablet formulation. All vertex points and one of the center edge points were replicated in order to get an estimate of the experimental variation, resulting in a total of 14 trials. The

Table 1.6 Design matrix for the effects of three components on tablet properties

Standard order	Lactose anhydrous (%)	MCC (%)	Lactose hydrous (%)	Response (hardness, kg)	Response (disintegration, min)
1	100	0	0	12.7	6.5
2	50	50	0	14.3	19.8
3	50	0	50	5.6	12.1
4	0	100	0	16.1	30.0
5	0	50	50	7.7	1.5
6	0	0	100	2.9	31.0
7	66.67	16.67	16.67	11.5	13.8
8	16.67	66.67	16.67	14.2	16.0
9	16.67	16.67	66.67	5.4	5.5
10	33.33	33.33	33.33	9.5	11.2
11	0	100	0	14.9	34.0
12	50	0	50	6.0	12.4
13	100	0	0	13.2	7.6
14	0	0	100	3.3	26.0

levels of the components are given in actual units, but since each blend also contains 0.5% magnesium stearate an exact statistical designation of the components is pseudocomponents. Two responses were monitored: tablet hardness and disintegration time, properties that frequently are in conflict and may indeed be difficult to reconcile.

Preparation of the blends, compression, and analysis of the tablets were carried out randomly. The settings of the tablet machine were identical in all cases. Notably, special care was exercised to employ the same tableting pressure. Results of model fitting and statistical computations afforded the results shown in Table 1.7.

Using the model selection criteria described earlier the quadratic model fits best for both responses, although the difference is marginal between the quadratic and special cubic models regarding tablet hardness. The corresponding contour plots are displayed in Figs. 1.8 (tablet hardness) and 1.9 (disintegration time).

The contour plot for hardness exhibits lines that are almost parallel, indicating few higher-order effects. Tablets containing hydrous lactose only are soft, whereas those made of pure MCC are very strong. Pure anhydrous lactose also furnishes tablets with excellent hardness.

By contrast, the contours of disintegration time display pronounced nonlinear (higher-order) effects. Tablets composed of MCC and hydrous

Table 1.7 Results of model fitting and statistical computations

	Hardness					
	ANOVA		**Lack of fit**			
Model	**F**	**p > F**	**F**	**p > F**	**Pred. R²**	**PRESS**
Linear	120.86	<0.0001	6.21	0.0484	0.9291	19.44
Quadratic	99.12	<0.0001	3.33	0.1354	0.9264	20.17
Special cubic	90.94	<0.0001	3.27	0.1412	0.8722	35.03
Cubic	Aliased – too few unique design points to determine all terms in this model					

	Disintegration					
	ANOVA		**Lack of fit**			
Model	**F**	**p > F**	**F**	**p > F**	**Pred. R²**	**PRESS**
Linear	2.58	0.1206	25.1	0.0038	−0.1260	1,571.93
Quadratic	30.00	<0.0001	2.34	0.2150	0.8381	225.95
Special cubic	24.20	0.0002	2.71	0.1795	0.5195	670.76
Cubic	Aliased – too few unique design points to determine all terms in this model					

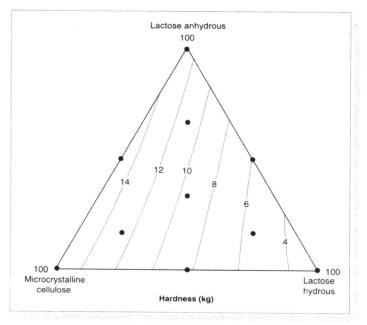

Figure 1.8 Contour plot for tablet hardness.

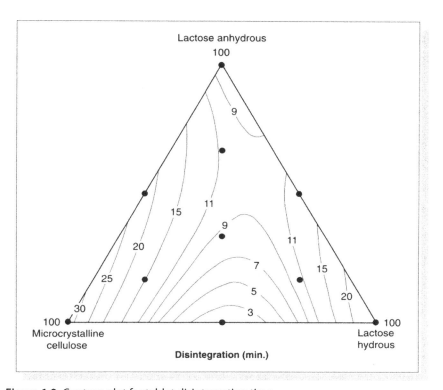

Figure 1.9 Contour plot for tablet disintegration time.

lactose in ca. 1:1 ratio have shortest disintegration time. Interestingly, tablets made of pure MCC and pure hydrous lactose disintegrate very slowly.

Combination (superimposing) of the two response surfaces can be used to find tablet compositions that fulfill given criteria. For instance, compositions satisfying hardness of more than 8 kg and disintegration time less than 5 min lie within the shaded area in Fig. 1.10.

To sum up, ASL design including only 14 trials results in seamless response surfaces furnishing complete estimates on the hardness and disintegration properties of tablets produced from *every conceivable composition* of the 3 direct compression materials. Of course, this would have been impossible by classical trial-and-error or one-factor-at-a-time approach. This fact demonstrates the enormous potential of the designed experimentation methodology.

There are several commercial software packages on the market dealing with statistical DOE and one of the best is Design-Expert from Stat-Ease Inc. (www.statease.com). The calculations and figures in this section were done with version 5.0.7 of the program.

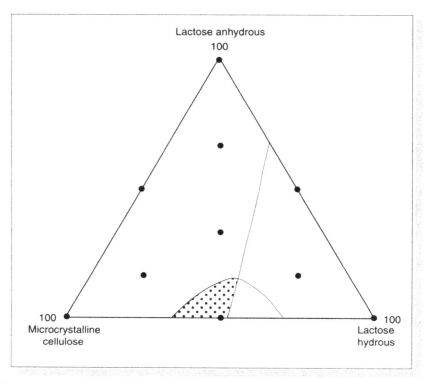

Figure 1.10 Superimposing of contour plots for hardness and disintegration time.

REFERENCES

[1] Augsburger LL, Hoag SW, editors. Pharmaceutical dosage forms: tablets. Unit operations and mechanical properties, vol. 1. 3rd ed. New York: Informa Healthcare; 2008.
[2] Augsburger LL, Hoag SW, editors. Pharmaceutical dosage forms: tablets. Rational design and formulation, vol. 2. 3rd ed. New York: Informa Healthcare; 2008.
[3] Liltorp K, Kristensen SL, Andresen T. Determination of particle sizes in the pharmaceutical industry. Copenhagen: Books on Demand; 2014.
[4] Rowe RC, Sheskey PJ, Cook WG, Fenton ME, editors. Handbook of pharmaceutical excipients. 7th ed. London: The Pharmaceutical Press; 2012.
[5] Eyjolfsson R. Mixing of pharmaceutical powders in tablet manufacture. Pharmazie 2001;56(7):590–1.
[6] Murphy TD. Design and analysis of industrial experiments. Chem Eng 1977;84(12): 168–82.
[7] Box GEP, Hunter WG, Hunter JS. Statistics for experimenters. An introduction to design, data analysis, and model building. New York: Wiley; 1978.
[8] Myers RH, Montgomery DC, Anderson-Cook CM. Response surface methodology: process and product optimization using designed experiments. 3rd ed. New York: Wiley; 2009.
[9] Cornell JA. Experiments with mixtures. Designs, models and the analysis of mixture data. 3rd ed. New York: Wiley; 2002.

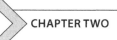

CHAPTER TWO

Conventional-Release (CR) Tablets

2.1 LOW-DOSE TABLET BY DIRECT COMPRESSION (DC)

2.1.1 Properties of active pharmaceutical ingredient (API)

White or almost white, crystalline powder. Freely soluble in water, in methylene chloride, and in methanol. pK_{a1} 3.7, pK_{a2} 9.8. Sensitive to oxidation. Batches with mean particle sizes, D[4,3], from 44 to 149 μm (laser light diffraction, dispersion Miglyol 812 + 10 s ultrasound) have been used.

2.1.2 Design

The composition of the tablets was based on information in *Repertorio Farmaceutico Italiano* of the originator's product that stated microcrystalline cellulose (MCC), corn starch, lactose monohydrate, and stearic acid as excipients. It was considered appropriate to employ DC excipients, i.e. Avicel PH-102, Tablettose 80, and Starch 1500, for adequate powder flow. Since Avicel PH-102 and Tablettose 80 are known to work best in DC formulations in the proportion 1:1 (see Fig. 1.10) this ratio was used in trial experiments with and without 11% Starch 1500. It was found that powder mixtures containing Starch 1500 had better compression properties, furnishing tablets (diameter 8 mm) with hardness of about 80 N and disintegration time of about 1 min. Dissolution was complete (100%) after 30 min (USP method, 0.01N HCl, 900 ml, paddles, 50 rpm; specification NLT 80% dissolved after 30 min).

Composition of tablets:

	mg/tablet	g/200,000 tablets	%
Active pharmaceutical ingredient (API)	25	5,000	13.9
Starch 1500	20	4,000	11.1
Avicel PH-102	65	13,000	36.1
Tablettose 80	65	13,000	36.1
Stearic acid 2236	5	1,000	2.8
Total	180	36,000	100

Design and Manufacture of Pharmaceutical Tablets. http://dx.doi.org/10.1016/B978-0-12-802182-8.00002-7

2.1.3 Manufacturing method

Avicel PH-102 and API were placed in this order in Collette-150 bowl and mixed (mixer-I, 150 rpm) for 60 s.

Avicel PH-102 and API were sieved through Comil 39R (1.0 mm).

API, Avicel PH-102, Starch 1500, and Tablettose 80 were placed in this order in Collette-150 bowl and mixed (mixer-I, 150 rpm) for 60 s.

Stearic acid 2236 was sieved through Comil 39R (1.0 mm) before weighing.

Stearic acid 2236 was placed on top of the mixture of API, Avicel PH-102, Starch 1500, and Tablettose 80, and mixed in Collette-150 (mixer-I, 150 rpm) for 45 s.

Flowability of powder mix was 15 mm (Flodex), which is good.

Tablet compression was performed with Manesty Betapress using 8 mm flat punches with break line at a speed of 50,000 tablets/h, which proceeded without any technical problems.

The product had a disintegration time of about 70 s and hardness of about 80 N. Friability was about 0.1% and coefficient of variation in determinations of content uniformity 1.6%. The manufacturing method was validated. A bioavailability investigation showed that the tablets were bioequivalent to the originator's product.

Packaged into Al/PVC blisters and cartons the tablets have a shelf life of 4 years at NMT 25°C.

2.1.4 Remarks

Since the API is freely soluble in water it is unlikely that its particle size will affect bioavailability.

However, particle size impacts flowability and content uniformity. An ideal particle size here is probably about 100 μm, corresponding to about $(1,000/100)^3 \times 25 = 25,000$ particles per tablet.

2.2 HIGH-DOSE TABLET BY DIRECT COMPRESSION

2.2.1 Properties of active pharmaceutical ingredient

White, crystalline powder. Sparingly soluble in water. Freely soluble in alcohol, very slightly soluble in methylene chloride. pK_a 9.5. Highly stable in solid dosage forms. The drug has very poor compaction properties.

2.2.2 Design

Due to the poor compression characteristics of the API a commercially available DC grade of it that contains 96% of active ingredient and 4% of povidone was used. Particle size specifications (sieving): NLT 20% retained on 100 mesh (149 μm) and NLT 70% retained on 270 mesh (53 μm). Two lubricants/glidants were used, i.e., magnesium stearate 0.5% and talc 4.5%. Three trial experiments were performed using: A, corn starch 16%; B, corn starch 8%/Avicel PH-102 8%; and C, Avicel PH-102 16% as diluents/binders/disintegrants. It was found that A furnished soft tablets with a short disintegration time, whereas C yielded a hard product with a long disintegration time. By contrast, B afforded tablets (7 × 19 mm capsule shaped) having acceptable values for these two important parameters, i.e., about 100 N and about 5 min, respectively. Dissolution was practically complete after 30 min [USP method, phosphate buffer (pH 5.8), 900 ml, paddles, 50 rpm; specification NLT 80% dissolved after 30 min].

Composition of tablets:

	mg/tablet	g/60,000 tablets	%
Active pharmaceutical ingredient DC grade, 96%	521	31,260	78.9
Corn starch	53	3,180	8
Avicel PH-102	53	3,180	8
Magnesium stearate 5712	3.3	198	0.5
Talc	29.7	1,782	4.5
Total	660	39,600	100

2.2.3 Manufacturing method

Corn starch and Avicel PH-102 were placed in Collette-25 bowl and mixed (mixer-I, 295 rpm) for 60 s.

Corn starch and Avicel PH-102 were sieved through Comil 39R (1.0 mm).

Corn starch/Avicel PH-102 premix and API were placed in this order in Collette-150 bowl and mixed (mixer-I, 150 rpm) for 90 s.

Magnesium stearate 5712 and talc were sieved through Comil 39R (1.0 mm) before weighing.

Magnesium stearate 5712 and talc were placed on top of the mixture of API, Avicel PH-102, and corn starch, and mixed in Collette-150 (mixer-I, 150 rpm) for 30 s.

Flowability of powder mix was 15 mm (Flodex), which is good.

Tablet compression was performed with Manesty Betapress using 7 × 19 mm capsule-shaped punches with break line at a speed of 25,000 tablets/h, which proceeded without any technical problems.

The product had a disintegration time of about 5 min and hardness of about 100 N. Friability was about 0.2% and coefficient of variation in determinations of mass uniformity 1.5%. The manufacturing method was validated. A bioavailability investigation showed that the tablets were bioequivalent to the originator's product.

Packaged into Al/PVC blisters and cartons the tablets have a shelf life of 5 years.

2.2.4 Remarks

Relatively high concentration of lubricant is necessary due to the poor compaction properties of the API.

2.3 LOW-SOLUBILITY API, LOW-DOSE TABLET BY WET GRANULATION (WG) [1]

2.3.1 Properties of active pharmaceutical ingredient

White or almost white, crystalline powder. Sparingly soluble in water, freely soluble in methanol. pK_{a1} 3.7, pK_{a2} 5.5. Very unstable in solid dosage forms if no precautions are taken. Main degradants are hydrolysis (HYD) and cyclization (CYC) products. Batches with mean particle sizes, D[4,3], from 6 to 22 μm (laser light diffraction, dispersion Tegiloxan 3 + 10 s ultrasound) have been used.

2.3.2 Design

Many drugs of this chemical group have been stabilized in tablets with alkaline excipients that defend against formation of CYC products, and by keeping moisture in the tablets low in order to minimize degradation via the HYD pathway. In this case, however, the originator had chosen another approach. According to information in *Repertorio Farmaceutico Italiano* it was found that these tablets contain hypromellose (HPM), MCC, pregelatinized starch, and sodium stearyl fumarate as excipients. Furthermore, it was discovered that this formulation/method was patented: the API is first coated with HPM followed by mixing with MCC and pregelatinized starch, lubrication with sodium stearyl fumarate, and compaction into tablets.

In view of this it was determined to employ stabilization with an alkaline excipient (sodium bicarbonate) but this was hampered by the fact that another patent precluded the use of monosaccharides and disaccharides as well as sugar alcohols as excipients. Therefore, calcium sulfate dihydrate (Compactrol) was selected as the main diluent, Starch 1500 (starch pregelatinized) as binder/disintegrant, and Pruv (sodium stearyl fumarate) as lubricant. Ethanol 96%/purified water (1 + 1) was chosen as granulation liquid in order to facilitate dissolution of the API in it, thus promoting reaction of the API with the stabilizator.

Small-scale experiments with Compactrol, Pruv, and Starch 1500 (5%, 10%, 15%, 20%, and 25%) showed that 10% Starch 1500 furnished the best tablets as to hardness, friability, and disintegration time. Additional trials using 1, 2, 3, 4, 5, or 6 mg of sodium bicarbonate per tablet containing 5 mg of API revealed that 5 mg of the stabilizator yielded tablets with the overall best chemical stability.

These tablets (5 × 10 mm capsule shaped) had hardness of about 60 N and disintegration time of about 40 s. Dissolution was almost complete (over 95%) after 30 min (based on a USP method, 0.1N HCl, 900 ml, paddles, 50 rpm; specification NLT 80% dissolved after 30 min).

Composition of tablets:

	mg/tablet	g/200,000 tablets	%
Active pharmaceutical ingredient (API)	5	1,000	1.9
Sodium bicarbonate	5	1,000	1.9
Compactrol	221.4	44,280	85.2
Starch 1500	26	5,200	10
Ethanol/purified water (1 + 1)	(56)	(11,150)	
Pruv	2.6	520	1
Total	260	52,000	100

2.3.3 Manufacturing method

All operations were carried out in an environmental relative humidity below 30%.

Sodium bicarbonate was milled in Apex J-5010 (0.25 mm), 2,240 rpm, hammers forward, before weighing.

Starch 1500, API, sodium bicarbonate, and Compactrol were placed in this order in Collette-150 bowl and mixed (mixer-I, 150 rpm, and chopper-I, 1,500 rpm) for 2 min.

Starch 1500, API, sodium bicarbonate, and Compactrol were sieved through Comil 39R (1.0 mm).

Starch 1500, API, sodium bicarbonate, and Compactrol were remixed in Collette-150 (mixer-I, 150 rpm, and chopper-I, 1,500 rpm) for 2 min.

Starch 1500, API, sodium bicarbonate, and Compactrol were granulated with ethanol 96%/ purified water (1 + 1), which was sprayed into the granulator bowl during 4 min (Collette-150, mixer-I, 150 rpm, and chopper-I, 1,500 rpm) followed by unaltered mixing speeds for further 1 min.

The granulate was sieved through Comil 375Q (9.5 mm).

The granulate was dried in Freund VFC-60 (220 l) fluid bed dryer for 40 min or until the granulate LOD was 0.75% (specification NMT 0.8%; Mettler HG-53, 80°C). Inlet air temperature was 55°C and maximum product temperature 43°C (specification NMT 45°C).

The dry granulate was sieved through Apex B-168 (1.0 mm), 2,240 rpm, knives forward.

Pruv was sieved through Comil 18R (0.5 mm) before weighing.

The sieved granulate was placed in 112 l tumbling mixer (GEI IBC), Pruv placed on top of it and mixed for 5 min at 12 rpm.

Flowability of finished granulate was 4 mm (Flodex), which is excellent.

Tablet compression was performed with Fette P2100 using 5 × 10 mm capsule-shaped punches with a speed of 90,000 tablets/h, which proceeded without any technical problems.

The product had a disintegration time of about 50 s and hardness of about 55 N. Friability was 0% and coefficient of variation in determinations of content uniformity 1.3%. The manufacturing method was validated. A bioavailability investigation showed that the tablets were bioequivalent to the originator's product. The manufacturing method was patented.

Packaged into Al/Al blisters and cartons the tablets have a shelf life of 2 years at NMT 25°C.

2.3.4 Remarks

Since the API is sparingly soluble in water it is conceivable that its particle size could affect dissolution/bioavailability. However, no problems pertaining to this have been encountered with API batches having mean particles sizes, D[4,3], from 6 to 22 μm (see above). An ideal mean particle size here is probably about 15 μm, corresponding to about $(1,000/15)^3 \times 5 = 1,500,000$ particles per tablet.

2.4 SOLUBLE API, LOW-DOSE TABLET BY WET GRANULATION

2.4.1 Properties of active pharmaceutical ingredient

White or almost white, crystalline powder. Soluble in water, sparingly soluble in methanol, practically insoluble in ethanol and in acetone. pK_{a1} 2.5, pK_{a2} 4.0. Relatively stable in solid dosage forms in the presence of slightly alkaline excipients. Main degradants are HYD and CYC products. Batches with mean particle sizes, D[4,3], from 5 to 50 μm (laser light diffraction, dispersion cyclohexane + 0.1% lecithin + 10 s ultrasound) have been used.

2.4.2 Design

Many drugs of this chemical group have been stabilized in tablets with alkaline excipients that defend against formation of CYC products, and by keeping moisture in the tablets low in order to minimize degradation via the HYD pathway. According to information in *Repertorio Farmaceutico Italiano* it was found that the originator's tablets contain calcium phosphate dibasic dihydrate (CPDD), mannitol, pregelatinized starch, and magnesium stearate as excipients. Apparently, the slightly alkaline properties (pH 7.4 in 20% aqueous slurry) of CPDD protect the drug against CYC. Furthermore, a primary aliphatic amino group in the drug's molecule may also help in this respect. On the other hand, this amino group precludes the use of excipients containing reducing saccharides (Maillard reaction).

Small-scale experiments with milled CPDD, 20% Mannitol 60 (mannitol), 0.7% magnesium stearate, and 5%, 10%, or 15% Starch 1500 (pregelatinized starch) using water as granulating liquid showed that 5% Starch 1500 provided tablets with adequate hardness but long disintegration time. Additionally, the granulate had very poor flowability. Therefore, unmilled CPDD (Di-Tab) was introduced as the main excipient. This resulted in a granulate with excellent flowability and tablets with good hardness but the disintegration time was still unsatisfactory. Consequently, 2%, 4%, or 6% of the superdisintegrant Ac-Di-Sol SD-711 (croscarmellose sodium) was added to the formulation and 4% of this excipient resulted in tablets with adequate hardness and disintegration time. Trial lots of these tablets (diameter 8 mm) had hardness of about 80 N and disintegration time of about 5 min. Dissolution was complete (100%) after 30 min (USP method, 0.1N HCl, 900 ml, paddles, 50 rpm; specification NLT 80% dissolved after 30 min).

Composition of tablets:

	mg/tablet	g/240,000 tablets	%
Active pharmaceutical ingredient (API)	5.45	1,308	2.6
Mannitol 60	42	10,080	20
Di–Tab	142.18	34,123.2	67.7
Starch 1500	10.5	2,520	5
Ac–Di–Sol SD-711	8.4	2,016	4
Purified water	(80)	(19,200)	
Magnesium stearate 5712	1.47	352.8	0.7
Total	210	50,400	100

2.4.3 Manufacturing method

Mannitol 60, API, Starch 1500, Ac-Di-Sol SD-711, and Di-Tab were placed in this order in Collette-150 bowl and mixed (mixer-I, 150 rpm, and chopper-I, 1,500 rpm) for 2 min.

Mannitol 60, API, Starch 1500, Ac-Di-Sol SD-711, and Di-Tab were sieved through Comil 32R (0.8 mm).

Mannitol 60, API, Starch 1500, Ac-Di-Sol SD-711, and Di-Tab were remixed in Collette-150 (mixer-I, 150 rpm, and chopper-I, 1,500 rpm) for 2 min.

Mannitol 60, API, Starch 1500, Ac-Di-Sol SD-711, and Di-Tab were granulated with purified water that was sprayed into the granulator bowl during 2 min (Collette-150, mixer-I, 150 rpm, and chopper-I, 1,500 rpm) followed by unaltered mixing speeds for further 2 min.

The granulate was sieved through Comil 375Q (9.5 mm).

The granulate was dried in Freund VFC-60 (220 l) fluid bed dryer for 90 min or until the granulate LOD was 1.9% (specification 1.5–3.0%; Mettler HG-53, 80°C). Inlet air temperature was 55°C and maximum product temperature 34°C (specification NMT 45°C).

The dry granulate was sieved through Apex B-168 (1.0 mm), 2,240 rpm, knives forward.

Magnesium stearate 5712 was sieved through Comil 18R (0.5 mm) before weighing.

The sieved granulate was placed in 112 l tumbling mixer (GEI IBC), magnesium stearate 5712 placed on top of it and mixed for 5 min at 12 rpm.

Flowability of finished granulate was 4 mm (Flodex), which is excellent.

Tablet compression was performed with Fette P2100 using 8 mm normal concave punches with break line. Tableting speed was 90,000 tablets/h, which proceeded without any technical problems.

The product had a disintegration time of about 5 min and hardness of about 55 N. Friability was 0% and coefficient of variation in determinations of content uniformity 1.5%. The manufacturing method was validated. A bioavailability study showed that the tablets were bioequivalent to the originator's product.

Packaged into Al/PVC blisters and cartons the tablets have a shelf life of 3 years at NMT 25°C.

2.4.4 Remarks

Since the API is freely soluble in water it is unlikely that its particle size will affect bioavailability.

However, particle size impacts content uniformity. But even a mean particle size of 50 μm (cf. properties of API above) would furnish about $(1{,}000/50)^3 \times 5.4 = 40{,}000$ particles per tablet, so this is hardly of any concern here.

2.5 LOW-SOLUBILITY API, HIGH-DOSE TABLET BY WET GRANULATION

2.5.1 Properties of active pharmaceutical ingredient

White or almost white, crystalline powder. Practically insoluble in water, soluble in ethanol (96%) and in methanol. pK_a 4.2. Stable in solid dosage forms. Batches with particle size about 50 μm and about 10 μm (optical microscopy of dry powders) have been used.

2.5.2 Design

According to information in *Repertorio Farmaceutico Italiano* the originator's tablets contain croscarmellose sodium, povidone, and magnesium stearate as excipients. Small-scale experiments were performed with API having 50 μm particle size (API-50 μm), 2%, 4%, or 6% croscarmellose sodium (Ac-Di-Sol SD-711), 4%, 6%, or 8% povidone, and 0.5% magnesium stearate using purified water as granulating liquid. It was found that 4% Ac-Di-Sol SD-711 and 6% povidone yielded excellent quality tablets (diameter 11 mm) having hardness of about 170 N and disintegration time about 7 min. By contrast, API-10 μm could not be granulated using this formulation. Granulation with ethanol 96% also gave unsatisfactory results. Consequently, this approach was abandoned.

Instead a formulation based on information in the literature was adopted. This encompasses use of 5.2% povidone as binder/wetting agent, 13.6% MCC (Avicel PH-102) as diluent, 4% sodium starch glycolate (Primojel) as disintegrant, and 0.2% magnesium stearate as lubricant. Granulation is performed with ethanol 96%. Trial lots having this composition furnished good quality tablets from both API-50 μm and API-10 μm. Hardness of the tablets (8.3 × 17 mm oval) was about 150 N and disintegration time about 5 min. Dissolution was complete (100%) after 45 min [USP method, 0.1 M phosphate buffer (pH 7.4), 900 ml, paddles, 50 rpm; specification NLT 80% dissolved after 45 min]. In fact, the two formulations are not very different except for the fact that the latter contains MCC. Therefore, it may be expected to be more forgiving with regard to the physical properties of the API.

Composition of tablets:

	mg/tablet	g/80,000 tablets	%
Active pharmaceutical ingredient (API-50 μm)	500	40,000	76.9
Povidone	34	2,720	5.2
Avicel PH-102	88.7	7,096	13.6
Primojel	26	2,080	4
Ethanol 96%	(180)	(14,400)	
Magnesium stearate 5712	1.3	104	0.2
Total	650	52,000	100

2.5.3 Manufacturing method

Avicel PH-102, API-50 μm, Povidone, and Primojel were placed in this order in Collette-150 bowl and mixed (mixer-I, 150 rpm, and chopper-I, 1,500 rpm) for 2 min.

Avicel PH-102, API-50 μm, Povidone, and Primojel were sieved through Comil 39R (1.0 mm).

Avicel PH-102, API-50 μm, Povidone, and Primojel were remixed in Collette-150 (mixer-I, 150 rpm, and chopper-I, 1,500 rpm) for 2 min.

Avicel PH-102, API-50 μm, Povidone, and Primojel were granulated with ethanol 96% that was sprayed into the granulator bowl during 4 min (Collette-150, mixer-I, 150 rpm, and chopper-I, 1,500 rpm) followed by unaltered mixing speeds for further 1 min.

The granulate was sieved through Comil 375Q (9.5 mm).

The granulate was dried in Freund VFC-60 (220 l) fluid bed dryer until the granulate LOD was 1.0% (specification NMT 1.1%, Mettler HG-53, 100°C). Inlet air temperature was 65°C and maximum product temperature 42°C (specification NMT 45°C).

The dry granulate was sieved through Apex B-46 (1.3 mm), 2,240 rpm, knives forward.

Magnesium stearate 5712 was sieved through Comil 18R (0.5 mm) before weighing.

The sieved granulate was placed in 112 l tumbling mixer (GEI IBC), magnesium stearate 5712 placed on top of it and mixed for 5 min at 12 rpm.

Flowability of finished granulate was 4 mm (Flodex), which is excellent.

Tablet compression was performed with Manesty Betapress using 8.3 × 17 mm elliptical/oval punches with break line. Tableting speed was 30,000 tablets/h, which progressed without any technical problems.

The product had a disintegration time of about 6 min and hardness of about 140 N. Friability was 0% and coefficient of variation in determinations of content uniformity 1.2%. A bioavailability study showed that the tablets were bioequivalent to the originator's product.

Packaged into Al/PVC blisters and cartons the tablets have a shelf life of 4 years.

2.5.4 Remarks

As shown the above manufacturing description refers to API with a particle size of 50 μm (API-50 μm). This method using the API-10 μm variety also provides good quality tablets but requires a considerable more amount of granulation liquid.

2.6 SOLUBLE API, HIGH-DOSE TABLET BY WET GRANULATION [2]

2.6.1 Properties of active pharmaceutical ingredient

Pale yellow, crystalline powder. Soluble in water, slightly soluble in methanol, very slightly soluble in ethanol, practically insoluble in acetone, in ethyl acetate, and in methylene chloride. pK_{a1} 6.3, pK_{a2} 8.5. Batches with mean particle size, D[4,3], about 100 μm (laser light diffraction, dispersant coconut oil) have been used.

2.6.2 Design

According to information in *Repertorio Farmaceutico Italiano* the originator's tablets contain MCC, crospovidone, corn starch, silicon dioxide colloidal, and magnesium stearate as excipients. Small-scale experiments were performed with 78% API, 19%, 17%, or 15% MCC (Avicel PH-102), 2%, 4%, or 6% crospovidone (Polyplasdone XL-10), 0.7% silicon dioxide colloidal (Aerosil 200), and 0.7% magnesium stearate using purified water as granulating liquid. Rather hard tablets with long and unacceptable disintegration times were obtained in all cases. Increasing the content of disintegrant (Polyplasdone XL-10) to 8% did not solve this problem either; the tablets (8 × 18 mm capsule shaped) obtained still disintegrated very slowly or in 12–15 min.

The disintegrant had been placed intragranularly in all the formulation experiments described above. Therefore, it was determined to place half of the disintegrant along with a portion of the diluent (Avicel PH-102) extragranularly (see composition of tablets below). The results were quite dramatic: the tablets (8 × 18 mm capsule shaped) obtained had a hardness of about 180 N and disintegration time of about 2 min! Dissolution was complete (100%) after 30 min (USP method, 0.01N HCl, paddles, 50 rpm; specification NLT 80% dissolved after 30 min).

Composition of tablets:

		mg/tablet	g/70,000 tablets	%
1	Active pharmaceutical ingredient (API)	582	40,740	77.6
2	Avicel PH-102	62	4,340	8.3
3	Polyplasdone XL-10	30	2,100	4
4	Purified water	(160)	(11,200)	
5	Avicel PH-102	36	2,520	4.8
6	Polyplasdone XL-10	30	2,100	4
7	Aerosil 200	5	350	0.7
8	Magnesium stearate 5712	5	350	0.7
Total		750	52,500	100

2.6.3 Manufacturing method

1 (Avicel PH-102), 2 (API), and 3 (Polyplasdone XL-10) were placed in this order in Collette-150 bowl and mixed (mixer-I, 150 rpm, and chopper-I, 1,500 rpm) for 2 min.

1 (Avicel PH-102), 2 (API), and 3 (Polyplasdone XL-10) were sieved through Comil 45R (1.2 mm).

1 (Avicel PH-102), 2 (API), and 3 (Polyplasdone XL-10) were remixed in Collette-150 (mixer-I, 150 rpm, and chopper-I, 1,500 rpm) for 2 min.

1 (Avicel PH-102), 2 (API), and 3 (Polyplasdone XL-10) were granulated with purified water that was sprayed into the granulator bowl during 4 min (Collette-150, mixer-I, 150 rpm, and chopper-I, 1,500 rpm) followed by unaltered mixing speeds for further 1 min.

The granulate was sieved through Comil 375Q (9.5 mm).

The granulate was dried in Freund VFC-60 (220 l) fluid bed dryer until the granulate LOD was 1.6% (specification NMT 2.0%, Mettler HG-53, 100°C). Inlet air temperature was 65°C and maximum product temperature 41°C (specification NMT 45°C).

The dry granulate was sieved through Apex B-82 (2.0 mm), 2,240 rpm, knives forward.

7 (Aerosil 200) was sieved through Comil 39R (1.0 mm) before weighing.

8 (magnesium stearate 5712) was sieved through Comil 18R (0.5 mm) before weighing.

The sieved granulate was placed in Collette-150 bowl, 5 (Avicel PH-102), 6 (Polyplasdone XL-10), and 7 (Aerosil 200) placed on top of it and mixed (mixer-I, 150 rpm) for 2 min.

8 (magnesium stearate) was placed on top of the granulate blend and mixed (Collette-150, mixer-I, 150 rpm) for 30 s.

Flowability of finished granulate was 10 mm (Flodex), which is good.

Tablet compression was performed with Manesty B3B using 8 × 18 mm capsule-shaped punches with break line. Tableting speed was 21,000 tablets/h, which proceeded without any technical problems.

The product had a disintegration time of about 1 min and hardness of about 180 N. Friability was 0.02% and coefficient of variation in determinations of mass uniformity 0.7%. The manufacturing method was validated. A bioavailability investigation showed that the tablets were bioequivalent to the originator's product.

Packaged into Al/PVC blisters and cartons the tablets have a shelf life of 3 years.

2.6.4 Remarks

Placing the disintegrant both intragranularly and extragranularly was of crucial importance in this case.

REFERENCES

[1] Eyjolfsson R. Calcium sulfate dihydrate: a useful excipient for tablets containing labile actives. Pharmazie 2004;59(9):725–6.
[2] Eyjolfsson R. Crospovidone: position in granulate and disintegration. Pharmazie 1999;54(12):945.

CHAPTER THREE

Slow-Release (SR) Tablets

3.1 SLOW-RELEASE TABLET USING A LIPOPHILIC RELEASE CONTROL AGENT

3.1.1 Properties of active pharmaceutical ingredient (API)

White or slightly yellowish, crystalline powder. Sparingly soluble in water, freely soluble in methanol, soluble in alcohol, slightly soluble in acetone. pK_a 3.8. Sensitive to oxidation. Batches with mean particle size, D[4,3], 7–34 μm (laser light diffraction, dispersion cyclohexane + 0.1% lecithin + 2 min ultrasonication) have been used.

3.1.2 Design

According to information in *Repertorio Farmaceutico Italiano* the originator's tablets contain cetyl alcohol as main release control agent. It was determined not to use this compound but to employ hydrogenated vegetable oil (Sterotex K) as this had already been utilized for the design of another slow-release (SR) tablet with good results.

Small-scale experiments were carried out with 16.7% API, 59.3%, 54.3%, 49.3%, or 44.3% lactose monohydrate (Pharmatose 150M), 15%, 20%, 25%, or 30% Sterotex K, 4% povidone, 0.5% magnesium stearate, and 4.5% talc using ethanol 96% as granulating liquid. It was found that the formulation with 25% Sterotex K afforded tablets whose dissolution profile was quite similar to that of the originator's product. A trial lot of this formulation furnished tablets (diameter 12 mm biconvex) with hardness of about 130 N and the following dissolution values: after 1 h 37.7%, after 4 h 72.9%, and after 7 h 92.7%. After manufacture of several trial lots and one pilot lot the following dissolution specifications were set: after 1 h 25–45%, after 4 h 60–80%, and after 7 h NLT 75% dissolved. Dissolution method: water, 900 ml, paddles, 50 rpm. Also, specification for target tablet hardness was set to 130 N (110–150 N).

Design and Manufacture of Pharmaceutical Tablets. http://dx.doi.org/10.1016/B978-0-12-802182-8.00003-9

Composition of tablets:

	mg/tablet	g/90,000 tablets	%
Active pharmaceutical ingredient (API)	100	9,000	16.7
Sterotex K	150	13,500	25
Pharmatose 150M	296	26,640	49.3
Povidone	24	2,160	4
Ethanol 96%	(55)	(4,950)	
Magnesium stearate 5712	3	270	0.5
Talc	27	2,430	4.5
Total	600	54,000	100

3.1.3 Manufacturing method

Pharmatose 150M, povidone, API, and Sterotex K were placed in this order in Collette-150 bowl and mixed (mixer-I, 150 rpm, and chopper-I, 1,500 rpm) for 2 min.

Pharmatose 150M, povidone, API, and Sterotex K were sieved through Comil 45R (1.2 mm).

Pharmatose 150M, povidone, API, and Sterotex K were remixed in Collette-150 (mixer-I, 150 rpm, and chopper-I, 1,500 rpm) for 2 min.

Pharmatose 150M, povidone, API, and Sterotex K were granulated with ethanol 96% that was sprayed into the granulator bowl during 4 min (Collette-150, mixer-I, 150 rpm, and chopper-I, 1,500 rpm) followed by unaltered mixing speeds for further 1 min.

The granulate was dried in Freund VFC-60 (220 l) fluid bed dryer until the granulate LOD was 0.3% (specification NMT 0.4%, Mettler HG-53, 100°C). Inlet air temperature was 65°C and maximum product temperature 44°C (specification NMT 45°C).

The dry granulate was sieved through Apex A-47 (2.7 mm), 2,240 rpm, knives forward.

Magnesium stearate 5712 and talc were sieved through Comil 18R (0.5 mm) before weighing.

The sieved granulate was placed in Collette-150 bowl, magnesium stearate and talc placed on top of it and mixed (mixer-I, 150 rpm) for 30 s.

Flowability of finished granulate was 16 mm (Flodex), which is good.

Tablet compression was performed with Manesty Betapress using 12 mm normal concave punches. Tableting speed was 22,000 tablets/h, which proceeded without problems.

The tablets had hardness of about 130 N. Friability was 0% and coefficient of variation in determinations of mass uniformity 0.6%. Dissolution results: after 1 h 38.0%, after 4 h 73.9%, and after 7 h 91.1% dissolved. The manufacturing method was validated. A bioavailability investigation showed that the tablets were bioequivalent to the originator's product.

Packaged into Al/PVC blisters and cartons the tablets have a shelf life of 3 years at NMT 25°C.

3.1.4 Remarks

Granulating with water was impossible due to the formation of an intractable sticky mass. There is slight tendency to picking/sticking to punches during tablet compaction like for other products of this type. This may be countered by using well-polished punches and by keeping the temperature in the tablet compaction cubicle low, preferably below 20°C. Particle size of API is critical and mean particle size, D[4,3], should be below 50 μm using the method outlined above. Tablets manufactured from batches of API outside this limit may fail to comply with the dissolution rate specification.

3.2 SLOW-RELEASE TABLET USING EUDRAGIT AND METHOCEL AS RELEASE CONTROL AGENTS

3.2.1 Properties of active pharmaceutical ingredient

White, crystalline powder. Sparingly soluble in water. Freely soluble in alcohol, very slightly soluble in methylene chloride. pK_a 9.5. Highly stable in solid dosage forms. The drug has very poor compaction properties.

3.2.2 Design

According to information in *FASS* (*Pharmaceutical Specialties in Sweden*) the originator's tablets contain paraffin and ethyl cellulose as release control agents. It was determined not to use this approach but to employ ammonio methacrylate copolymer type B (Eudragit RS PO) and hypromellose 2208 (Methocel K100M Premium) as there is much information in the literature about these excipients.

Due to the poor compression characteristics of the API a commercially available direct compression grade of it that contains 96% of active and 4% of povidone was used. Particle size specifications (sieving): NLT 20% retained on 100-mesh (150 μm) and NLT 70% retained on 270-mesh (53 μm) screen. Small–scale experiments were carried out with tablets containing 521 mg API, 40 mg Eudragit RS PO, 15 mg talc, 4 mg magnesium stearate, and 80, 100, or 120 mg Methocel K100M Premium using ethanol 96% as granulating liquid. It was discovered that the formulation with 100 mg Methocel K100M Premium furnished tablets with a dissolution curve that was practically superimposable on that of the originator's tablets. A trial lot of this composition yielded tablets (7 × 19 mm capsule shaped) with hardness of about 100 N and the following dissolution values: after 1 h 11.8%, after 4 h 28.8%, after 8 h 44.0%, after 12 h 55.5%, and after 18 h 70.5% dissolved. Following manufacture of several trial lots and one pilot lot the following dissolution specifications were adopted: after 1 h 5–20%, after 4 h 20–40%, after 8 h 35–55%, after 12 h 45–65%, and after 18 h 60–80%. Dissolution method: water, 1,000 ml, baskets, 50 rpm. Baskets must be used; otherwise the tablets will stick to the bottom of the dissolution vessels giving erroneous results. Specification for tablet hardness was set to 90–140 N.

Composition of tablets:

	mg/tablet	g/80,000 tablets	%
Active pharmaceutical ingredient DC grade, 96%	521	41,680	76.6
Methocel K100M Premium	100	8,000	14.7
Eudragit RS PO	40	3,200	5.9
Ethanol 96%	(180)	(14,400)	
Magnesium stearate 5712	4	320	0.6
Talc	15	1,200	2.2
Total	680	54,400	100

3.2.3 Manufacturing method

Methocel K100M Premium and Eudragit RS PO were placed in Collette-150 bowl and mixed (mixer-I, 150 rpm) for 2 min.

Methocel K100M Premium and Eudragit RS PO were sieved through Comil 45R (1.2 mm).

Methocel K100M Premium and Eudragit RS PO were remixed in Collette-150 (mixer-I, 150 rpm) for 2 min.

API was placed on top of Methocel K100M Premium and Eudragit RS PO, and mixed in Collette-150 (mixer-I, 150 rpm) for 2 min.

API, Methocel K100M Premium, and Eudragit RS PO were granulated with ethanol 96% that was sprayed into the granulator bowl during 2 min (Collette-150, mixer-I, 150 rpm).

The granulate was sieved through Comil 375Q (9.5 mm).

The granulate was dried in Freund VFC-60 (220 l) fluid bed dryer until the granulate LOD was 1.2% (specification NMT 1.4%, Mettler HG-53, 100°C). Inlet air temperature was 65°C and maximum product temperature 42°C (specification NMT 45°C).

The dry granulate was sieved through Comil 75R (1.9 mm).

Magnesium stearate 5712 and talc were sieved through Comil 18R (0.5 mm) before weighing.

The sieved granulate was placed in Collette-150 bowl, magnesium stearate and talc placed on top of it and mixed (mixer-I, 150 rpm) for 30 s.

Flowability of finished granulate was 4 mm (Flodex), which is excellent.

Tablet compression was performed with Manesty Betapress using 7 × 19 mm capsule-shaped punches. Tableting speed was 22,000 tablets/h, which proceeded without any problems.

The tablets had hardness of about 120 N. Friability was 0.1% and coefficient of variation in determinations of mass uniformity 0.5%. Dissolution results: after 1 h 12.3%, after 4 h 29.2%, after 8 h 44.9%, after 12 h 56.9%, and after 18 h 71.5% dissolved. The manufacturing method was validated. A bioavailability study showed that the tablets were bioequivalent to the originator's product.

Packaged into Al/PVC blisters and cartons the tablets have a shelf life of 5 years.

3.2.4 Remarks

Granulating with water was impossible due to gel formation. Relatively high concentration of lubricant is necessary due to the poor compaction properties of the API.

3.3 SLOW-RELEASE TABLET USING A MIXTURE OF METHOCELS AS RELEASE CONTROL AGENT [1]

3.3.1 Properties of active pharmaceutical ingredient

White or almost white, crystalline powder. Practically insoluble in water, soluble in ethanol (96%) and in methanol. pK_a 4.2. Stable in solid dosage forms. Batches with particle size about 50 μm and about 10 μm (optical microscopy of dry powders) have been used. Many batches of the 10-μm quality have been analyzed by laser light diffraction using dispersion in water + 5 drops 1% Nonidet + 30 s ultrasound. This has given mean particle sizes, D[4,3], from 16 to 21 μm.

3.3.2 Design

According to information in *Repertorio Farmaceutico Italiano* the originator's tablets contain only two excipients, i.e., a small amount of hypromellose 2208 as release control agent and magnesium stearate as lubricant. It was also discovered that this formulation was patented. Initial small experiments along these lines showed that the API-10 μm could not be granulated with water and the other (API-50 μm) furnished tablets with large and unacceptable variations in the dissolution data. Moreover, the supplier of API-50 μm ceased to deliver it. In view of this and a high risk of patent infringement this approach was discontinued.

It was considered likely that inclusion of a soluble excipient (lactose monohydrate = Pharmatose 150M) in the formula, utilization of binder (povidone), use of two grades of hypromellose 2208 (Methocel K100LV and Methocel K4M), and ethanol 96% as granulating liquid would solve both the technical and the patent obstacles. Eight trial lots were prepared containing 69.4% API-10 μm, 5% povidone, 15% Pharmatose 150M, and 0.5% magnesium stearate. Various ratios of Methocel K100LV and Methocel K4M were included in the tablets for release control as shown in the following percentages: 10/0, 7.5/2.5, 5/5, 4.4/5.6, 3.75/6.25, 3.1/6.9, 2.5/7.5, and 0/10.

It was found that the formulation with 3.75% Methocel K100LV and 6.25% Methocel K4M furnished tablets with a smooth dissolution curve that was practically superimposable on that of the originator's product. Therefore, the following preliminary dissolution specifications were set: at 1 h 5–20%, at 4 h 25–45%, at 8 h 45–65%, at 12 h 60–80%, and at 18 h NLT 80%. Dissolution method: simulated intestinal fluid without enzymes (pH 7.5, USP), 900 ml, baskets, 50 rpm. Baskets must be used; otherwise the tablets will stick to the bottom of the dissolution vessels giving erroneous results.

Composition of tablets:

	mg/tablet	g/7,000 tablets	%
Active pharmaceutical ingredient (API-10 μm)	500	3,500	69.4
Methocel K100LV Premium	27	189	3.75
Methocel K4M Premium	45	315	6.25
Povidone	36	252	5
Pharmatose 150M	108.4	758.8	15.1
Ethanol 96%	(225)	(1,575)	
Magnesium stearate 5712	3.6	25.2	0.5
Total	720	5,040	100

3.3.3 Manufacturing method

API-10 μm, Methocel K100LV Premium, Methocel K4M Premium, povidone, and Pharmatose 150M were placed in this order in Collette-25 bowl and mixed (mixer-I, 295 rpm and chopper-I, 1,500 rpm) for 2 min.

API-10 μm, Methocel K100LV Premium, Methocel K4M Premium, povidone, and Pharmatose 150M were sieved through Comil 39R (1.0 mm).

API-10 μm, Methocel K100LV Premium, Methocel K4M Premium, povidone, and Pharmatose 150M were remixed in Collette-25 (mixer-I, 295 rpm and chopper-I, 1,500 rpm) for 2 min.

API-10 μm, Methocel K100LV Premium, Methocel K4M Premium, povidone, and Pharmatose 150M were granulated with ethanol 96% that was sprayed into the granulator bowl during 2 min (Collette-25, mixer-I, 295 rpm and chopper-I, 1,500 rpm) followed by unaltered mixing speeds for further 2 min.

The granulate was sieved through Comil 375Q (9.5 mm).

The granulate was dried in GEA T2 (60 l) fluid bed dryer until the granulate LOD was 0.7% (specification NMT 1.0%, Mettler HG-53, 100°C). Inlet air temperature was 65°C and maximum product temperature 44°C (specification NMT 45°C).

The dry granulate was sieved through Apex B-82 (2.0 mm, 2,240 rpm, knives forward).

Magnesium stearate 5712 was sieved through a 0.18 mm hand sieve before weighing.

The sieved granulate was placed in Collette-25 bowl, magnesium stearate placed on top of it and mixed (mixer-I, 295 rpm) for 30 s.

Flowability of finished granulate was 16 mm (Flodex), which is good.

Tablet compression was performed with Manesty B3B using 8 × 18 mm capsule-shaped punches. Tableting speed was 21,000 tablets/h, which proceeded without any problems.

The tablets had hardness of about 240 N. Friability was 0% and coefficient of variation in determinations of mass uniformity 0.3%. Dissolution results (coefficient of variation expressed in percent in parentheses): after 1 h 11.7% (2.2), after 4 h 31.1% (0.6), after 8 h 52.3% (1.3), after 12 h 71.1% (1.6), and after 18 h 95.4% (1.1) dissolved. The tablets were packaged into HDPE containers and put on stability trial at 25°C/60% relative humidity (RH) and at 40°C/75% RH for 0, 1, 3, and 6 months. They were found to be chemically and physically stable. Dissolution rate did not change at 25°/60% RH and only insignificantly at 40°/75% RH.

3.3.4 Remarks

Scale-up, validation, and bioavailability studies were not carried out on this formulation due to lack of commercial interest. This author feels confident that these matters would have proceeded with elegance.

REFERENCE

[1] Eyjolfsson R. Hydroxypropyl methylcellulose mixtures: effects and kinetics of release of an insoluble drug. Drug Dev Ind Pharm 1999;25(5):667–9.

INDEX

Printed in the United States
By Bookmasters